MY MENOPAUSAL METAMORPHOSIS

How my change of life, gave the boot to societal strife

Written by Elaine Jones

Illustrated by Lana Lee

First Hardcover edition April 2022
First Paperback edition April 2022

Book design by Lana Lee

ISBN: 978-0-578-36751-4 (hardcover)

Published by Lainey's Logic LLC
www.laineyslogic.com

Have you ever spent a day questioning everything you do?

Why do you cross your legs or dye your hair? Do you even have a clue?

One day I sat and wondered were my actions all my own.

Or had they been influenced by an entity unknown?

Was it family or friends who intervened in Mother Nature's plan?

Was it religion, education, or interference from The Man?

I decided to take a journey down memory lane.

To see if my actions could somehow be explained.

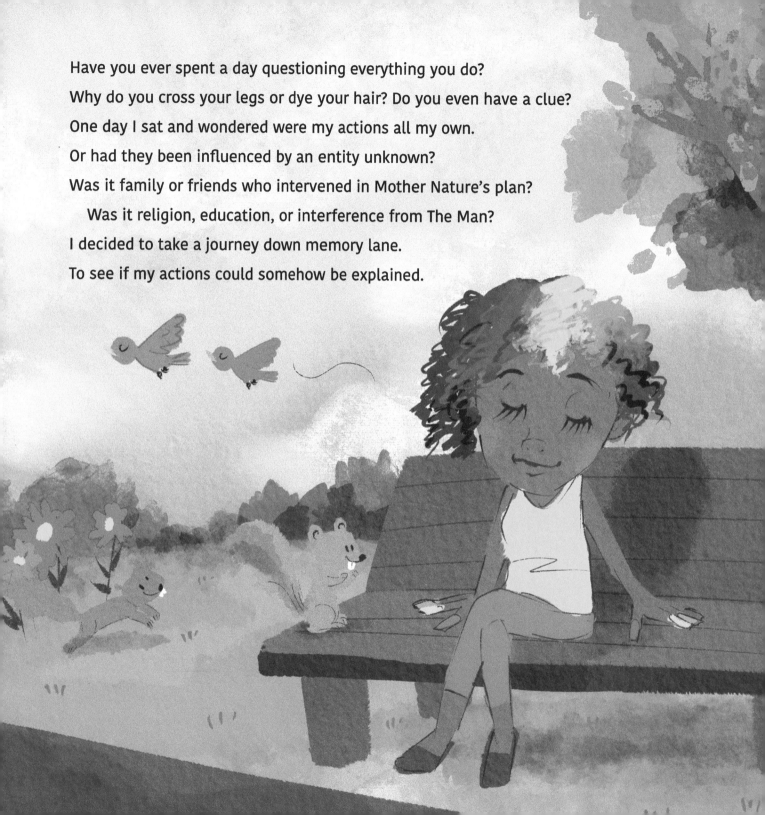

It all began while still in my mother's womb.

Societal norms had dictated how I should be groomed.

Yes, you heard me right; this was all planned before my birth.

Society had decided what would be my worth.

This "worthy" formula is based on things for which I have no control.

Like my race, sex, location, or spiritual soul.

Who are my parents, and how were they bred?

What their occupation is (if any). What kind of life had they led?

How can I control this? Are they blind? Can't they see?

I was born just this morning, bright and early at 2:03.

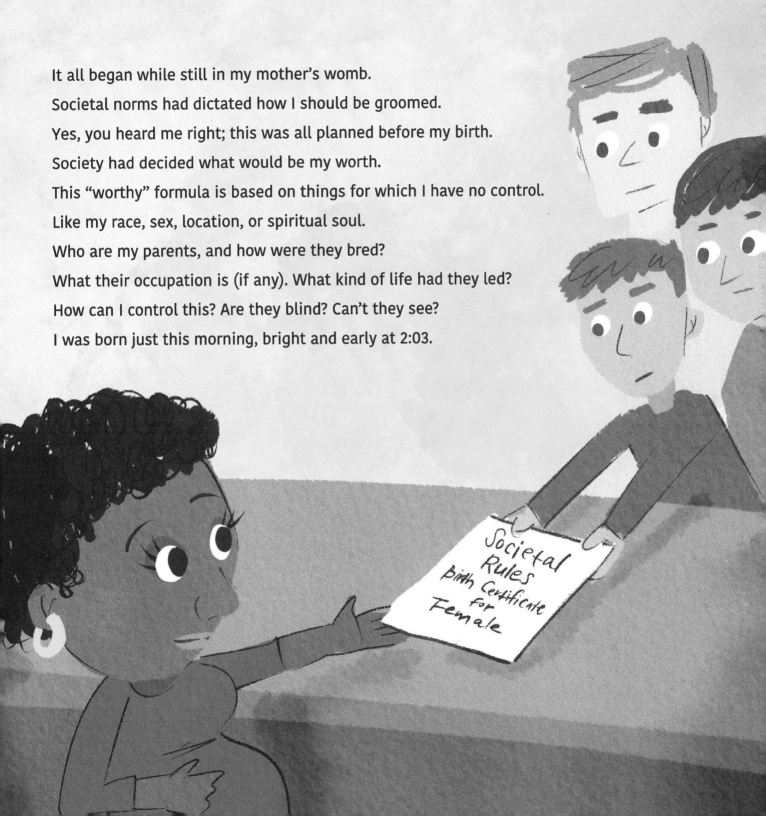

Born into this world as a female was mistake number one.

I'm expected to be subordinate to someone born as a son.

As a child, I am adorned in pink with ribbons and curls in my hair.

White shoes and a dress must fit perfectly, or people will stare.

I grow from an infant into a toddler and question everything in sight.

What's this, what's that, hmm that doesn't seem quite right.

Because as a child, I move about using only my instincts.

Which is an innate survival mechanism; no need to think.

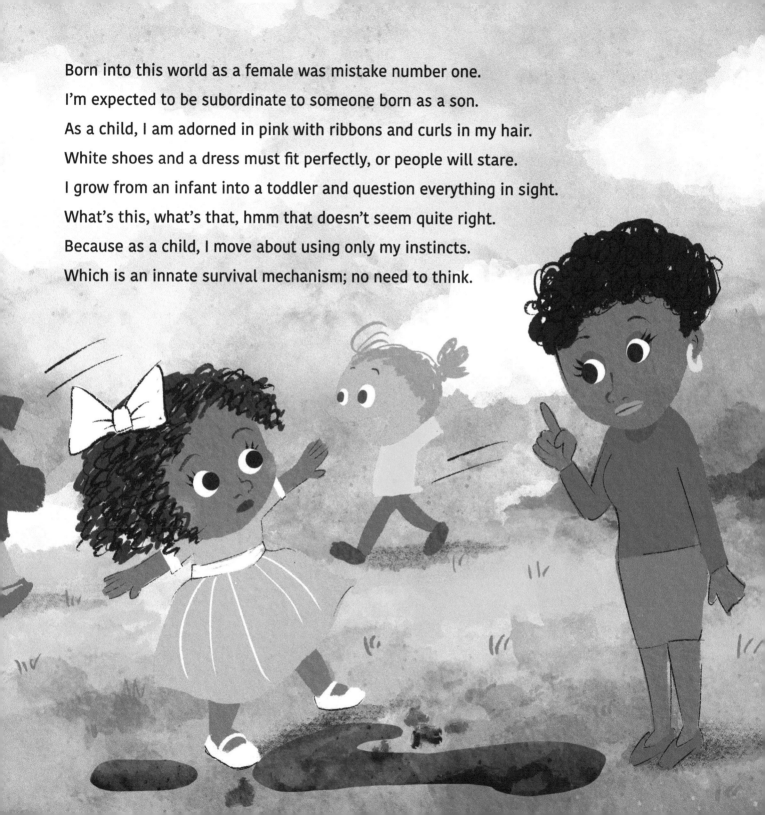

By age five, society demands that it's time I attend school.

I am given a curriculum, a set of things to do.

My teachers advise me how to play, sit, stand, and walk.

How to read, write, spell, and the correct way to talk.

For twelve years or more, I am told how to think.

And slowly but surely, I begin to ignore my instincts.

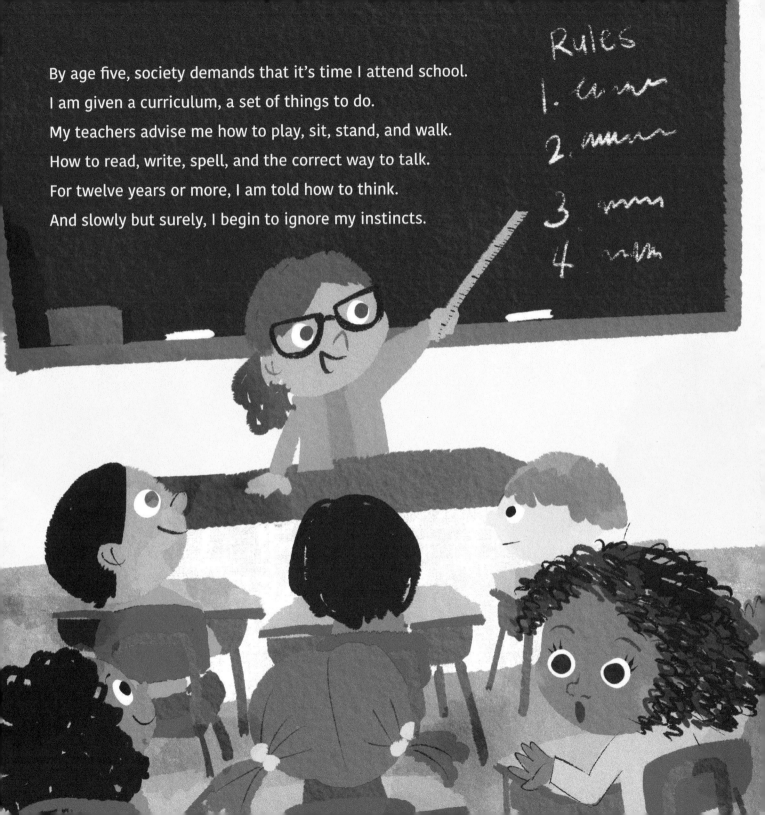

I begin to conform in everything I do.

From the clothing I wear to the music I listen to.

I start to act, look, and feel like the Connecticut wives.

I'm like the people who drank the juice and lost their lives.

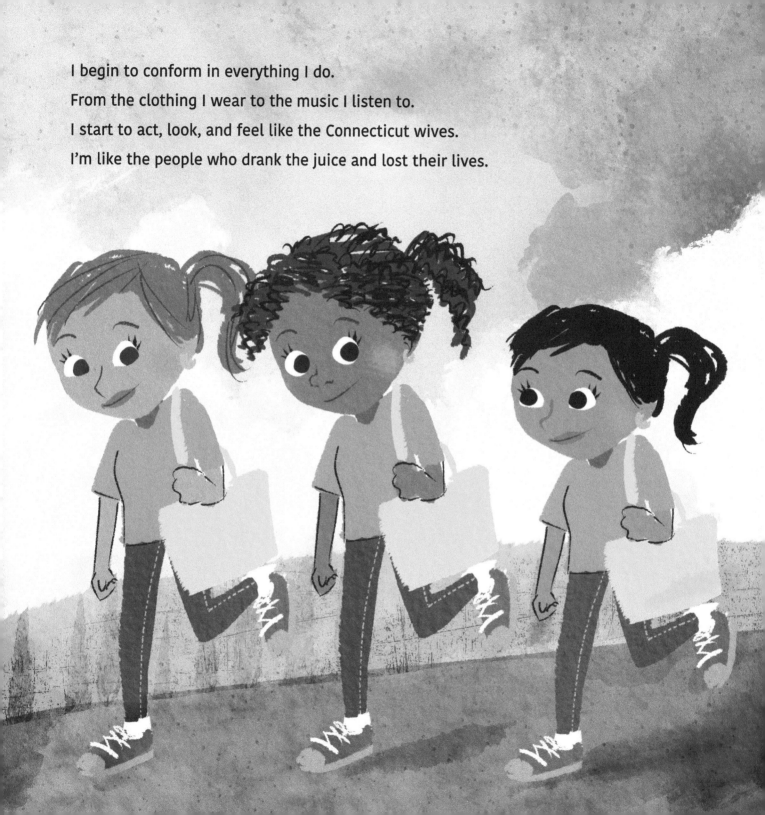

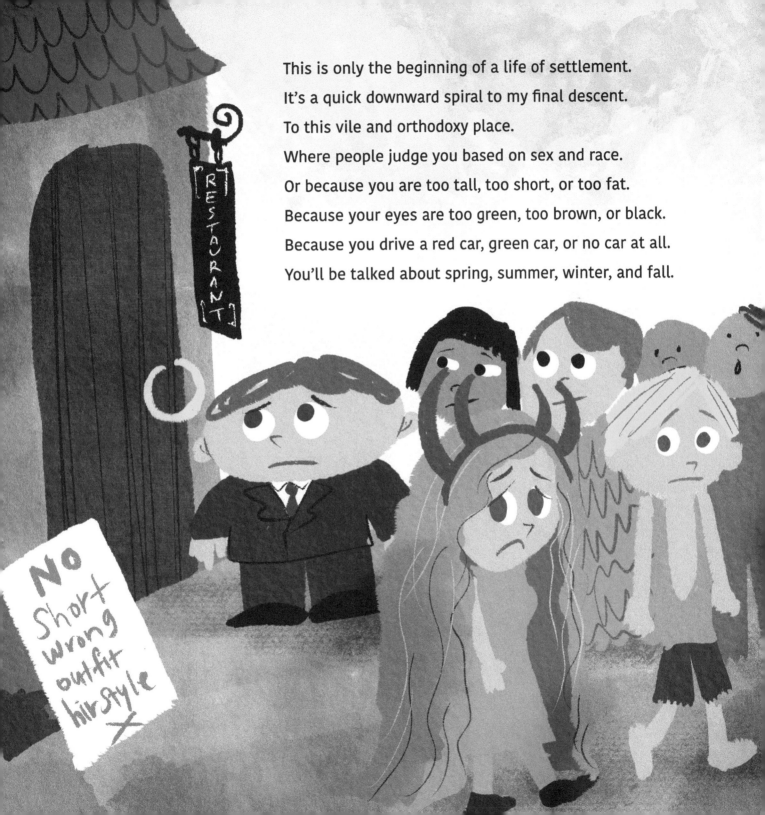

This is only the beginning of a life of settlement.

It's a quick downward spiral to my final descent.

To this vile and orthodoxy place.

Where people judge you based on sex and race.

Or because you are too tall, too short, or too fat.

Because your eyes are too green, too brown, or black.

Because you drive a red car, green car, or no car at all.

You'll be talked about spring, summer, winter, and fall.

Next, on to college, where I'm brainwashed while being charged big bucks.

As I train for a job that might make me self-destruct.

I prepared for a hot job needing qualified people right away.

Guess what? That job is obsolete by the time I reach graduation day.

You see, trade schools that taught you how to produce things with your hands

were shut down; experts stated in the future, there was be no demand.

How cretinous is that? What experts created that false vision?

You will always need a seamstress, a plumber, an electrician!

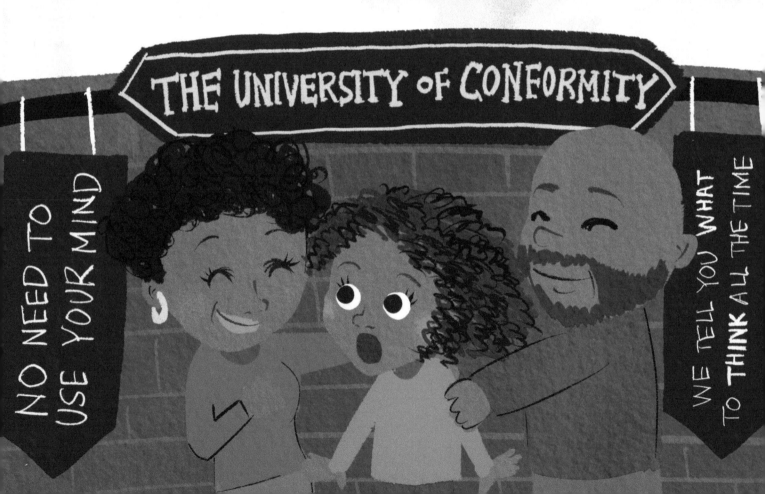

Now I'm saddled with student loan debt that makes no sense at all.

And I can't find a job, not even at the mall.

I take on several gigs to try and pay at least some of my debt.

I'm depressed, just plain miserable, and begin to fret.

I know this is not good for my mental or physical well-being.

I don't like what I do, how I feel, or what I am seeing.

Still, I continue on this path for decades to come.

Because everyone I know is doing it, I'm not the only one.

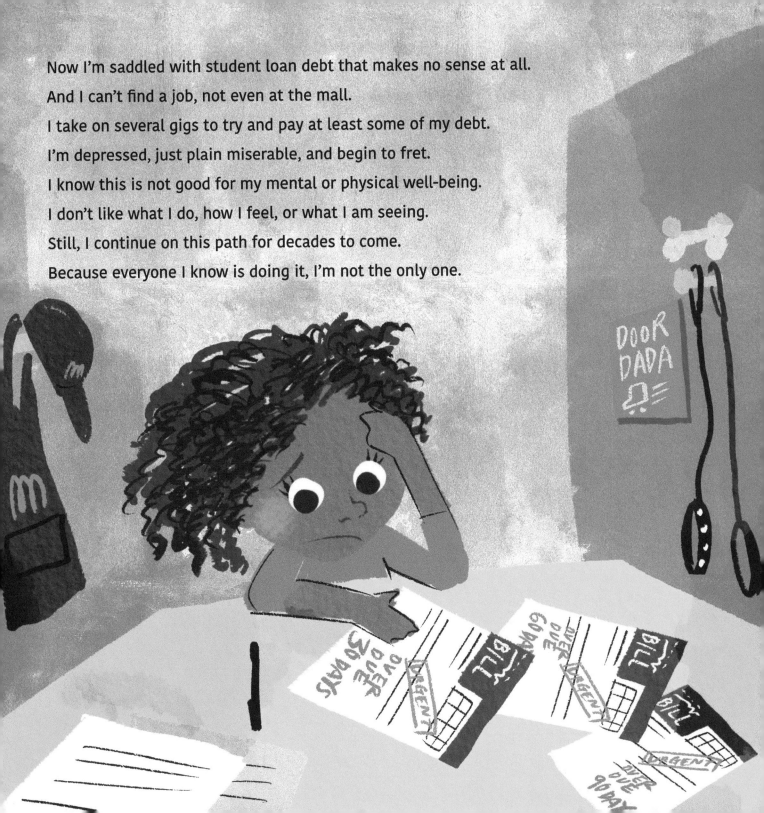

Everywhere I look, people have settled.
Settled for a job, settled for a house.
Settled for a salary, settled for a spouse.
Settled for a friend, settled for a clothing size.
Everyone has compromised.

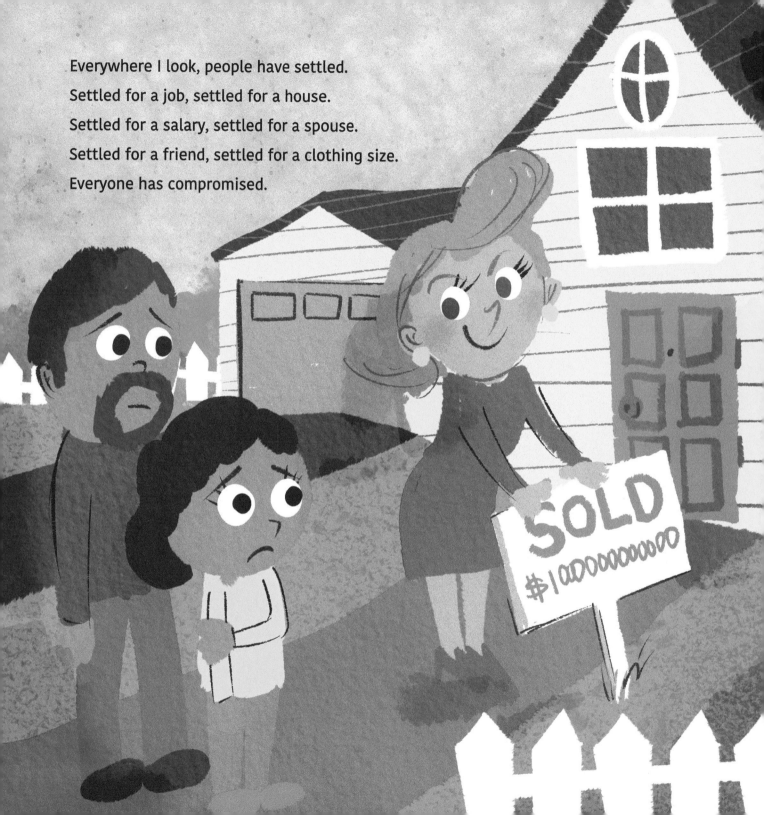

As the years go by, it's time to draw the line.

Incorrectly, I listened to society but not my own body and mind.

My body's been nudging me, providing signs all along.

Telling me to stop what I am doing it's not right; this is wrong.

For all these decades, I've turned, and I've bent.

Only to please others in a bad environment.

There have been many warning signs and many hints.

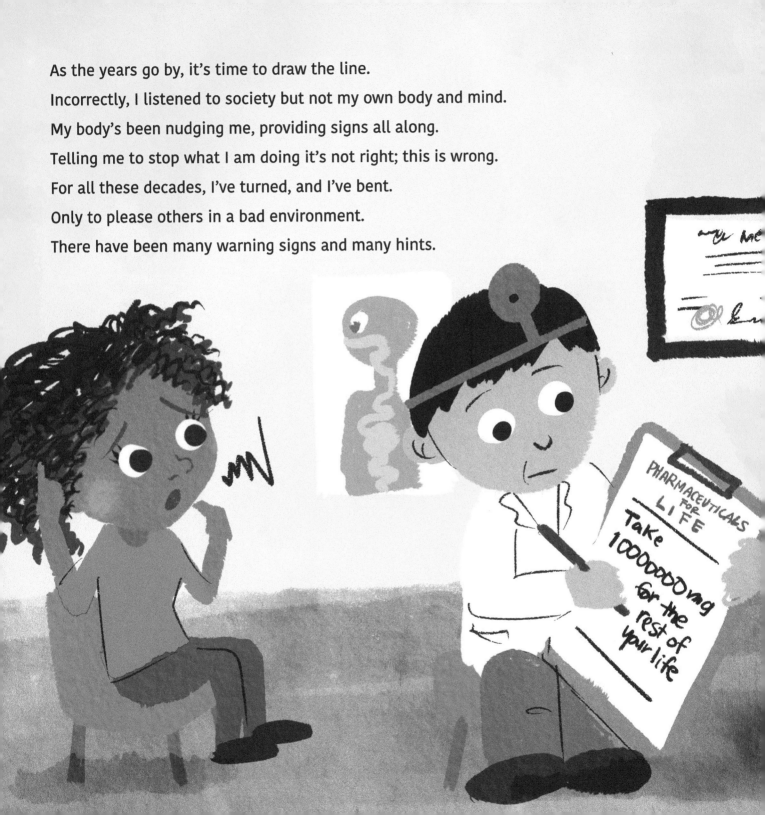

Then late one evening, a little past the fifth decade of my life,

while reading a book about injustice, crime, and civil rights.

A storm began brewing, causing hail and a severe downpour.

The wind blew profusely and shook my front door.

The lights started to flicker and filled me with dread.

I ran to get my flashlight, tripped over my cat, fell BOOM! Bumped my head.

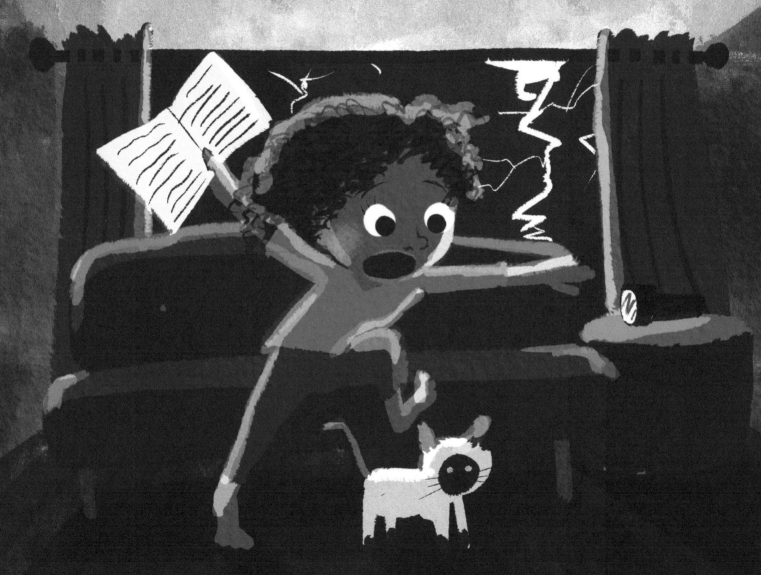

When I came to, I looked up and saw something I will never forget.

And until this day, I have never again seen something like it yet.

It was a hologram of a black woman dressed in armor from head to toe.

I stood up and instinctively knew what this meant for sure.

It was the time in life when you had to put on your big girl drawers.

Yes, it was finally time, time for the pause...

Menopause.

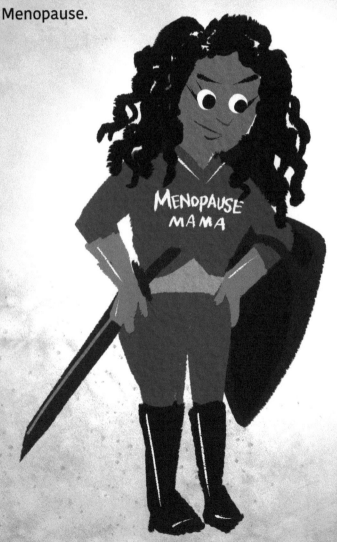

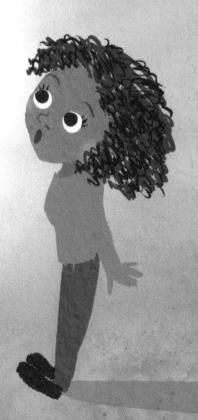

I had heard so much about it from when I was young.

But everything I heard was terrible, and nothing about it was fun.

Oh, the pain, oh the anger, the forgetfulness, and the sweats.

Oh, the weight gain, hair loss, and shopping at outlets.

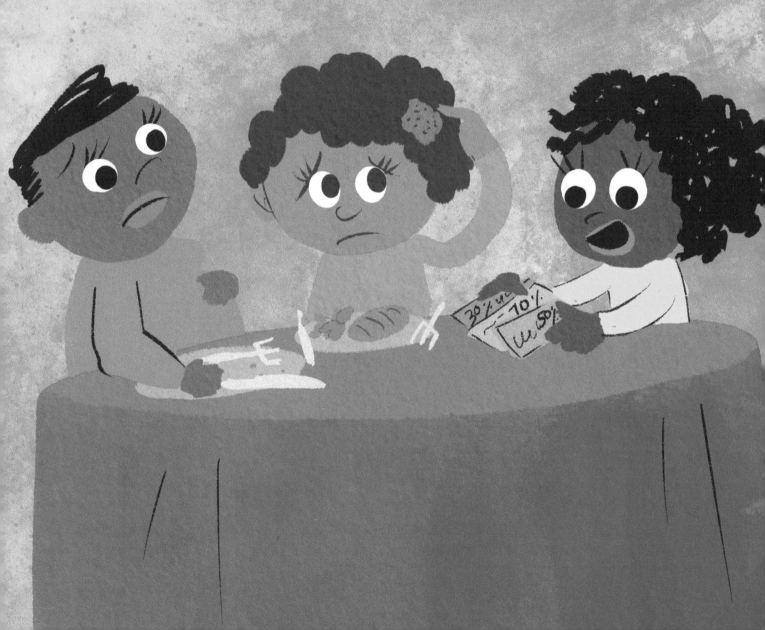

But my experience was different from anything I had heard.

It was nothing like the trauma my friends told me would occur.

It was a joyous occasion and an excellent experience for me.

Just like the verse in "Amazing Grace," I once was blind, but now I see.

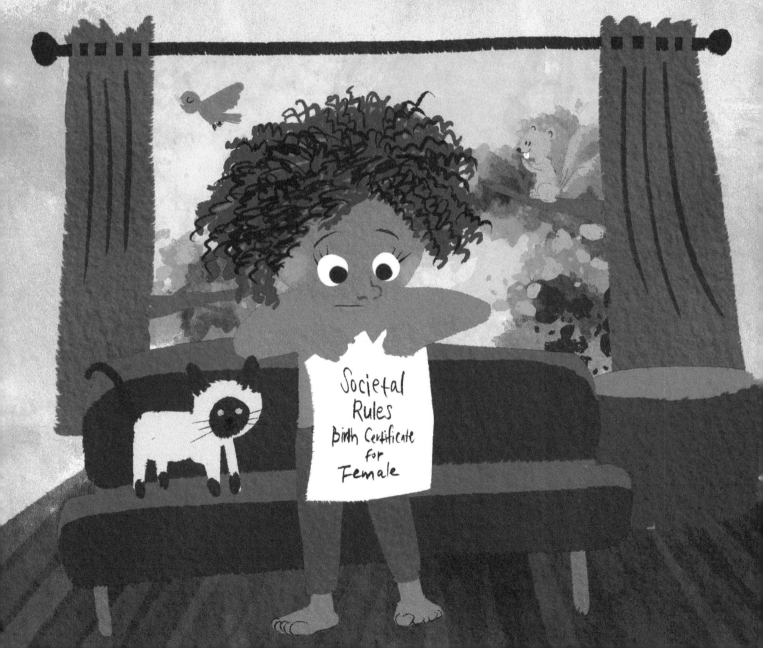

BING! A bell went off inside of my mind.

I knew I must leave conformity behind.

No longer would I or could I go against my own body's desire.

I would become focused and do only as I aspired.

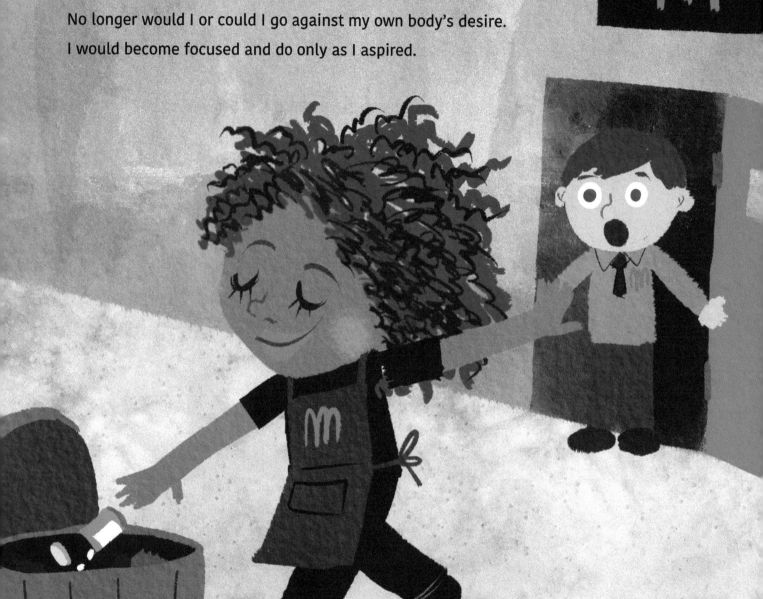

This change of thought was a new form of inspiration.
My body and mind's sole purpose are self-preservation.
Why'd it taken so long for me to figure it out?
Society's involvement in my business, no doubt.

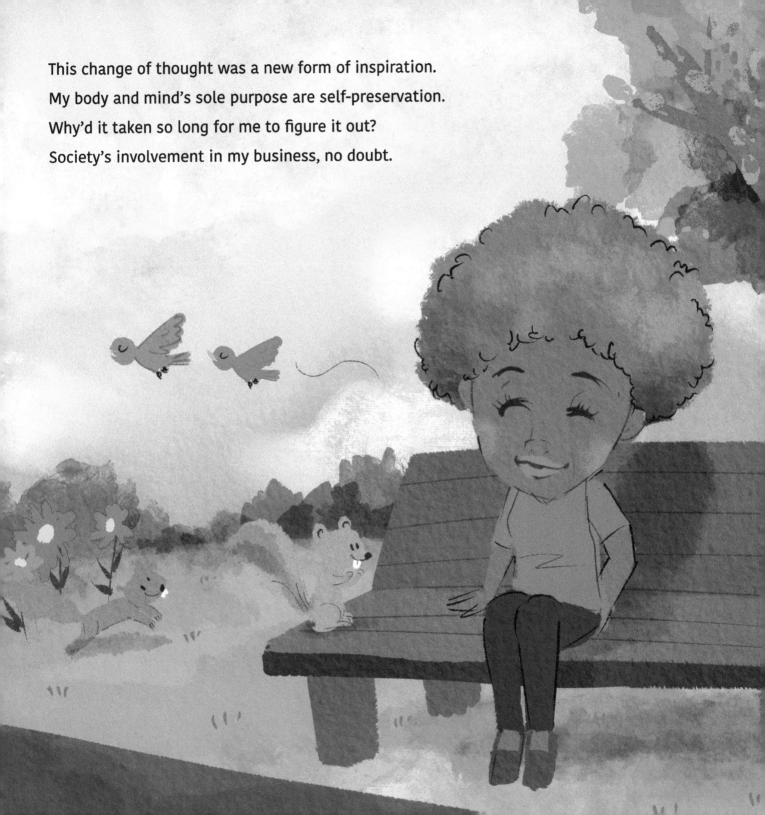

All the signs my body provides are for my good.

Unlike external factors such as that fine young man from my hood.

Every woman will reach this plateau, naturally or by force.

It's a part of the life cycle. You get it, don't you? Of course.

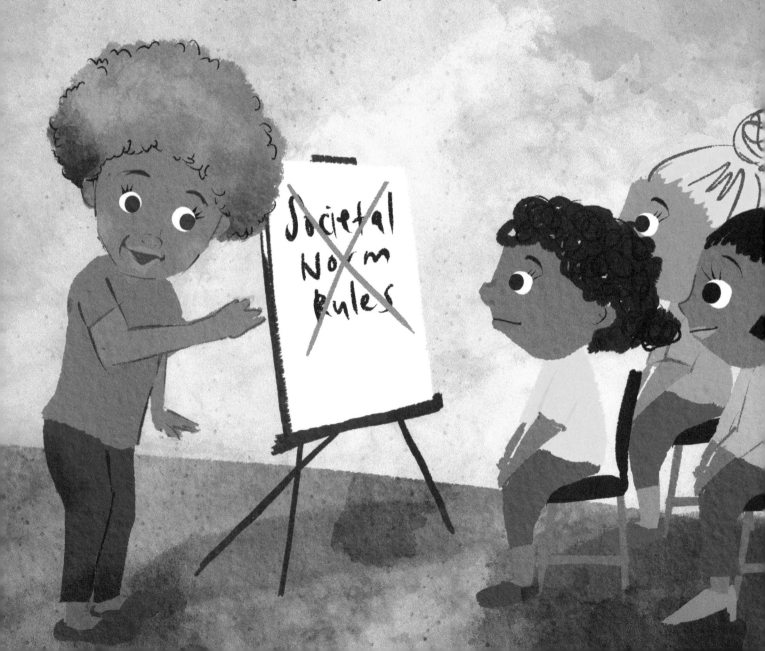

So, please don't get upset and focus on despair.

Because you think your breast will reach your derriere.

There is a whole lot you can do in advance to prepare.

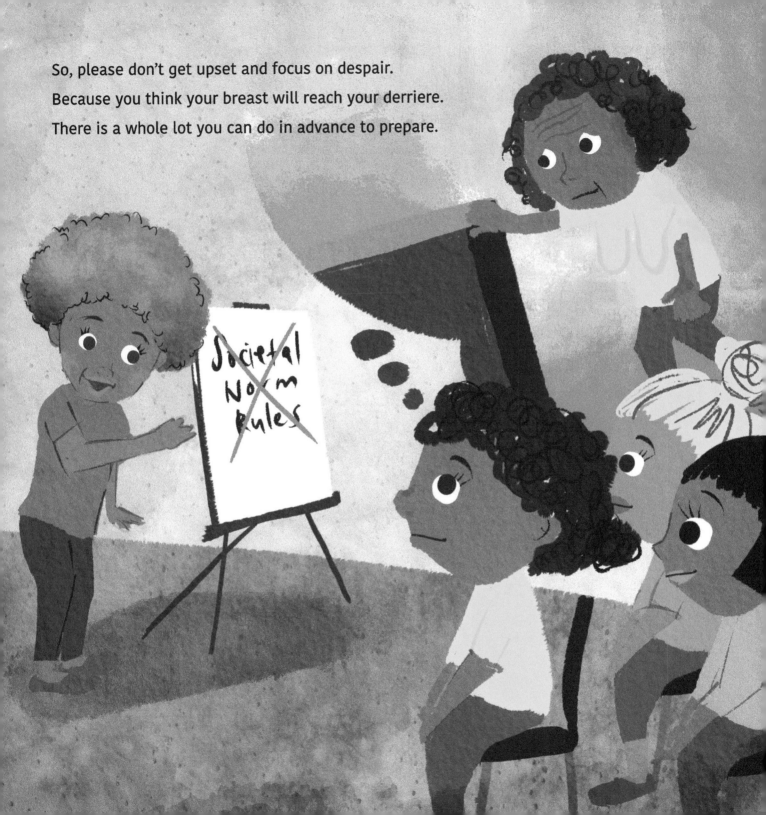

There are lessons to be learned if we just look deep.

The final phase of this journey can bring you comfort and peace.

Acceptance of oneself is the name of the game.

There is no one else like me, is what you can claim.

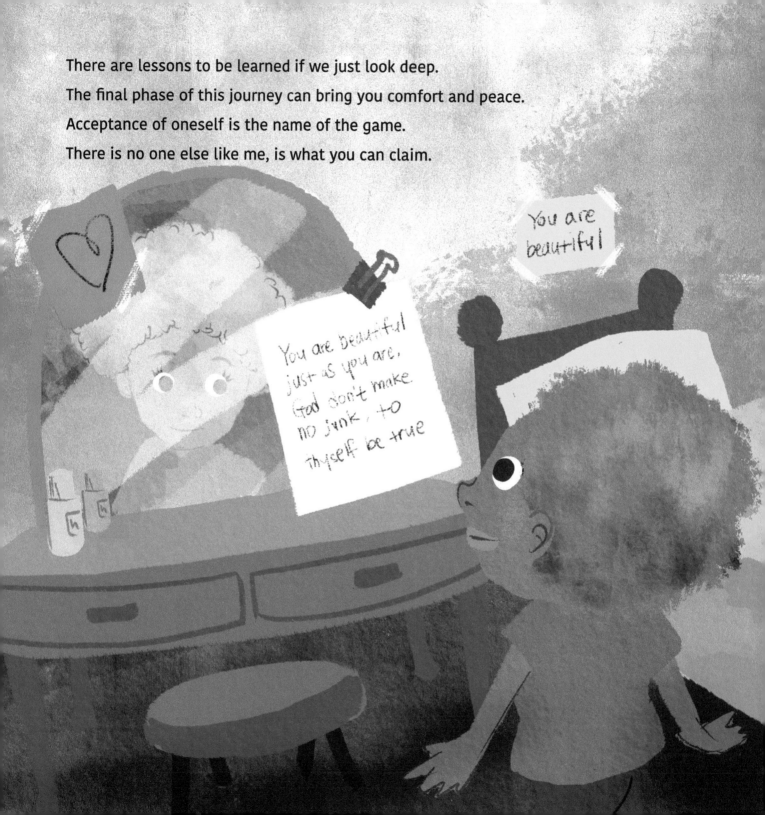

Never stop questioning the actions you take.

Let your life lessons be self-made mistakes.

Keep yourself mentally, spiritually, emotionally, and physically fit.

Be cautious with your incredible life and limit what you permit.

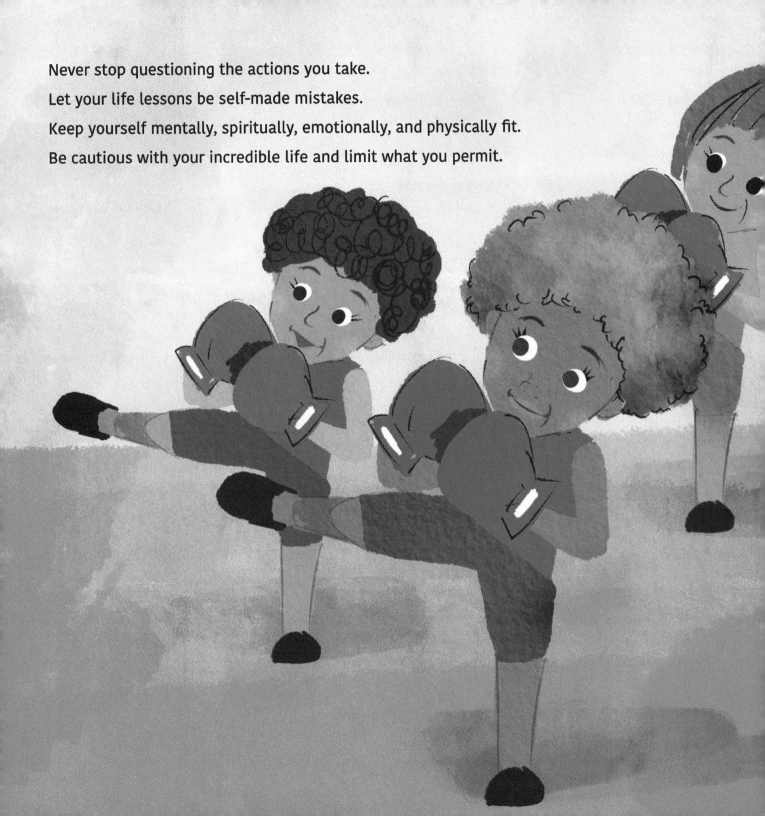

Be wise while you are young and question all you've been told.

You have but one life, live it well, live it bold!

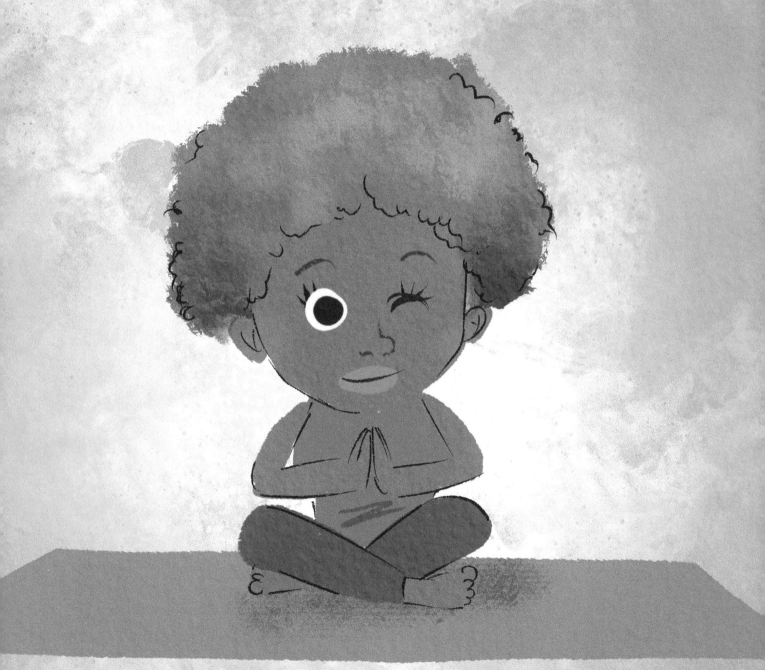

DEDICATION

This book is dedicated to the Matriarchs of my life, Aunts: Elaine, Laura, Nell, Phyllis, Mable, Sally, Kitty, Mrs. Anderson, Ms. Mendez, Dot, Mother, Haunt, Rochelle, Loretta, and Masita; thank you for your guidance, wisdom, knowledge and tough love. I love you all.

My sister-cousins Renee, Denise, Kay-Kay, Maia, Aisha, Tyniqua, Dachelle, and Jasmine. Thank you for your friendship, support, encouragement, and laughter. I love you all.

To the Salcedo and Jones clan, thank you for the conversations, parties, and laughter; how you all make me laugh. I've gained many beautiful, talented, funny brothers, sisters, nieces, and nephews. Too many to name, I love you all dearly.

To my children gained through marriage, Tervell, Khrystal, and Travis, thanks for allowing me to be a part of your life and sharing your dad with me. I love you all.

To my nieces and nephews, Jasmine, Dachelle, Deron, Vito, Ramel, Malik, Rochelle, and Chase, God has truly blessed me with your presence. You help to balance me with your kind and calm demeanors. I love you all very much.

To my Girlz Tina, Silvia, Cindy, Cheryl, Jackie, Crystal, Rita, Stella, Lisa, and Callie, thank you all for the many years of friendship through good and bad times.

To my son Daron, you make me think, laugh, and learn. The student is now the teacher. Thank you for accepting and loving me with all of my faults. To Linette, thank you for your caring and kind demeanor and for being a wonderful mother to Jayleen. Thank you to my granddaughter, Jayleen, for providing this family with a future. I pray that you follow your internal path and settle for nothing but the best. I love you all immensely.

To those who have gone on to glory: Granddaddy, thank you for always being that ever-present male figure in my life and teaching me our family history. To Mommy, thank you for giving me life, for providing an internal flame in me that seems never to go out, and for having been a wonderful, caring, and giving person. To my Big Bro, how I miss your presence, love, guidance, and wisdom. Thank you for always being my protector and teacher. To Rochelle, I often think of how our relationship from childhood to womanhood was beginning to blossom. I miss your beauty, style, and determination.

To my wonderful husband, Bruce, thank you for this long, funny, scary, bumpy, and wonderful journey. Thank you for your "never back down, stand up for what you believe in" demeanor. For your ability to stay calm under pressure and think on your feet. For your spontaneity and how you never cease to amaze me with some of the comments that come out of your mouth. Thank you for always making me laugh. My love for you continues to grow.

Finally, I dedicate this book to my God for bringing me through many trials and tribulations and giving me the strength to go on and make a way out of no way. For loving me more than I've sometimes loved myself. Thanks for allowing me yet another day to be the best I can be.

CPSIA information can be obtained
at www.ICGtesting.com
Printed in the USA
BVHW020952050522
636222BV00007B/121